Simplest Diet Ever

ISBN   978-0-9559781-0-4

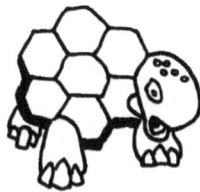

Simplest Diet Ever

Kathy Robinson

Dedication

for

Ja, Tim, and Si

Grateful thanks to
Kent Anderson for the cartoons
James Robinson for the cover and logo
Ros Rogers for proof reading the final draft
Vikki, Lisa, and Linda for being encouraging
Nicola, Monika, and Klaus for editorial assistance

SIMPLEST DIET EVER

Contents

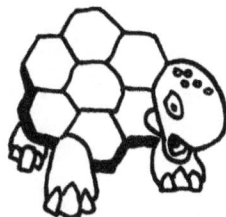

Chapter 1

Simplest diet ever

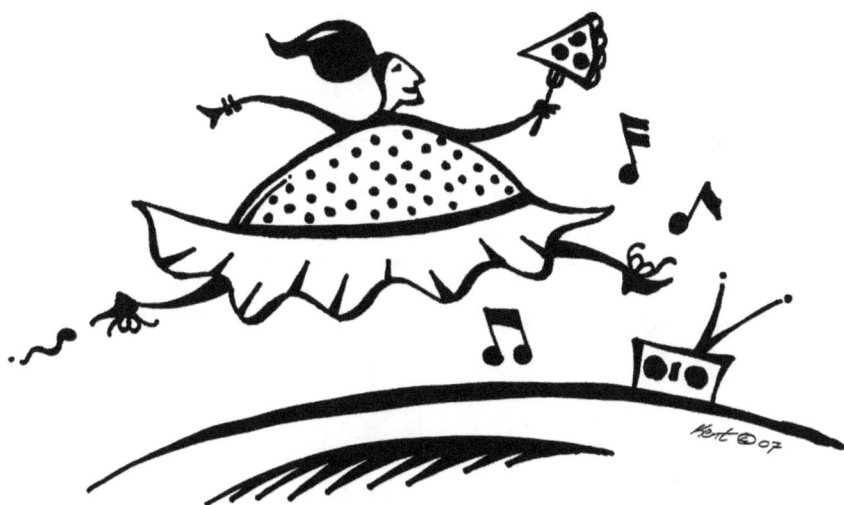

Eat less, move more

There couldn't be a simpler diet!
EAT LESS *and* MOVE MORE

Food is the body's money. When we eat it is rather like depositing money into a bank account. A lot of people have a current account at the bank, post office or building society. We deposit money into it, and use it for our everyday needs and expenses. Some people also have a savings account where they keep money aside and accumulate it. We might put money into our saving account occasionally, or on a regular basis. In fact we can instruct the bank to transfer surplus money from the current into the savings account.

There are two ways to reduce the amount of money in the savings account. The first is to stop paying into it. The second is to dip into the savings to meet your everyday expenses. So you stop paying in, and you start taking out.

The money and the bank accounts are a picture to help us understand what is going on in our body when we eat. If we eat more than we need the remainder gets stored up in a fat savings account. I hear you saying that some people can eat just what they like and never put on any weight at all. That is absolutely true, grossly unjust, extremely unfair, but true. Some of us have very efficient bodies and don't need to eat as much, and we find it easier to save for a rainy day.

Some of us have been building up our fat saving account for years, slowly, steadily putting a little aside on a regular basis. Others have had some sort of windfall that has boosted their savings.

Just as a bank can change the exchange rate or the interest rate, so our bodies change the amount they need for day to day use, and the saving arrangements over time. Middle age

9

spread is not a low fat margarine! It's a change in the interest rate.

So, how does the body use food? It's rather like a car and fuel. Food is the body's fuel. We need other things, like water and air too. But we definitely need food! Some cars run on unleaded petrol, others on diesel. Some people have different diets because of preference, availability, medical condition, religious or cultural beliefs. Lots of us have been on a 'weight reducing' diet, and some of us have even lost weight on it. Others of us have lost our tempers, our patience, our self-esteem, and even the will to live!

We can lose weight if we EAT LESS *and* MOVE MORE. Let's stop saving up for a rainy day, and instead spend more. We do this by eating less than our body needs, and by moving our bodies more.

It's sounds so simple doesn't it? Simple, but not easy. If it were easy we wouldn't all have shelves full of diet books and still be fat. If it were easy we would be able to keep off those pounds, and stones, that we have shed only for it to creep back on.

As a society we see the weight issue as the problem, rather than considering that it might be the result of a problem. Perhaps you know someone, who is struggling with their weight, who has never got over a bereavement, illness, separation, rejection, abuse, loss of a relationship or status or job. It is often much easier to make these connections for other people, whilst being oblivious to our own behaviour. I am not suggesting that we will ever be quite the same again.

You may have heard the word 'holistic' used in terms of a medical treatment plan. It means to consider the whole person, and not just the weight, or the trauma or the illness. So let's do that with overeating. Let's consider ourselves as a whole person without disconnecting the fat bits from the

10

rest. In fact lets go further and say that these fat bits are part of me!

Sometimes we say jokingly that there's a thin person in me waiting to get out. There's just one person, and this person is waiting to get thin. It'll be a long wait, unless we accept that only one person can do something about it!

Perhaps you think of yourself as no more than a body in front of the mirror. But look again, is there no heart? No mind? No longings or soul? Be open to new challenges in all areas of your life as a whole person. Take up the quest to EAT LESS *and* MOVE MORE. After all, what have you got to lose?

Quick quiz
Just answer YES or NO and total each column

DO YOU	YES	NO
Get up in the night and raid the fridge?		
Eat frozen food, too desperate to defrost it?		
Wait until you are alone to eat and eat?		
Feel that the food controls you?		
Buy a meal for two and eat it alone?		
Shop for food pretending it's for someone else?		
Buy food items as gifts, but never give them?		
Eat the children's chocolate or sweets?		
Have a collection of diet books?		
Have a thin person inside waiting to come out?		
Think it's unfair that some can eat what they like?		
Lose weight only to put it back on again?		
Feel bad about yourself because you are fat?		
Find it hard to buy clothes?		
Have a wardrobe full of clothes that don't fit?		
Dread finding clothes suitable for social events?		
Feel ashamed of your body?		
TOTAL		

How did you get on?

SCORE   YES 0 – 2

- You are reading the wrong book!

or

- You intended to read for someone else and have not been honest with your own answers. Bravely read on!

or

- You are reading the book so that you can help other people.

SCORE   YES 3 – 5

- Perhaps you have put on weight because you have just been eating slightly too much over a long period of time, or not made an adjustment for middle age. You are not a food addict, but you do relate to some of the issues. This book is for you, so stick with it!

or

- You are just reading the book so that you can help other people. Be open to finding something for yourself as well. The fact that you do relate to some of the issues will make it easier for you to understand and help those who relate to many of them.

SCORE   YES 6 – 10

- Thank you for being honest. You do have food issues, and you are reading the right book for you

or

- You are just reading the book so that you can help other people. You have probably had a bit of a shock then. Perhaps you have never realised that you yourself have some issues relating to food. Or perhaps you think you can't face them. This book will help you help others, but it will also help you if you'll let it.

SCORE   YES 11 – 17

- You are reading the right book. Be encouraged, because admitting where you are starting from is the best place to start. You have already taken an important step. You have chosen to be honest, and I admire you for that. Thank you for having the courage to read this book. You can move forward.

or

- You are just reading the book so that you can help other people. It's very unlikely that you will be able to help other people with their food issues if you are not facing up to your own. If you don't want to get sorted then why not give this book to someone that does? Think very carefully over this decision. You are looking at the possibility of turning your life around. Do you want to throw that away?

So, you want to EAT LESS *and* MOVE MORE. If you want to stop putting on weight, you have to stop saving up in your fat account. You want to use up some of those savings so for that you need to be more active.

We need to start making choices. Dealing with addictive behaviour is often much more complex than making a simple choice to stop. Yo-yo dieting is clear evidence of this. People lose amazing amounts of weight only to put it all, and maybe more, back on. Been there, done that! Why do we want to do that? Of course we don't, but we can't stop ourselves.

Four out of five people, in the UK, who have lost a lot of weight put it all back on again. Many know all there is to know about being on a diet, but just can't maintain the necessary changes to their long term eating patterns.

Just focusing on our eating habits isn't the whole answer. We will be exploring other facets of wellbeing in our more holistic approach to the complex issues that affect our body weight. How ever many other issues need sorting on the way, we are aiming towards being able to EAT LESS *and* MOVE MORE.

Are you waiting for the crunch? The lists of what you can and can't have and the system for counting up what you have? I hope you won't be disappointed, because that is not coming. All weight-reducing diets basically work in the same way. However they are labelled and marketed, and however you add up what you are having, they work because they help you to EAT LESS.

If you have a medical condition please get a check up from your Doctor before you start. Some of the information in this book may not apply to you so please be guided by the Doctor. If you have never been on a diet before, or not done exercise for years then a check up is also advisable.

14

When some people try and follow a set diet plan they find that they are focusing on food all the time, and they end up eating more. If you relate to that then simply EAT LESS of the food you normally eat. Try not to lower your fruit and vegetable intake but reduce anything else.

A set plan is just a tool that helps some people to EAT LESS. If you are interested in a plan you will find information in Chapter 2, otherwise skip straight past it.

If you have followed one particular diet several times before you may find that it is less effective each time you go back to it. The body is amazing and it has all sorts of automatic protective systems. When it thinks there isn't going to be enough food around it hangs on to every last store it can to give you the best chance of survival during a siege. If you have taught it to recognise one particular diet it will do just that, and dig it's heels in only giving up it's fat supply as a last resort. So try something different.

It is ok to leave food on your plate. Some of us are from the 'clear your plate' generation. If you eat the food it's gone. If you put it in the bin it's gone. Either way it's gone. Even if your parents made you feel guilty by reminding you about starving children in Africa, you can't actually send your last few cold soggy vegetables to them. If you want to help, EAT LESS and send the money you save on your grocery bills. If you are full, give yourself permission to stop eating.

To get our bodies to use up our fat stores we need to MOVE MORE. If you are waiting with dread for me to say gym sessions you are in luck. If you are comfortable in the gym then that's a great way to exercise. But if your heart sinks at the mention of the word then that's not the place for you.

You can go to a class if you want to, but all I am recommending is that you MOVE MORE. Look for ways of adding additional movement into your everyday life. You could hide the television remote control. How about moving things around in your kitchen? Instead of the kettle, mugs, spoons and coffee all being together, move something so that you have to walk around to get them.

Try a television free day, or a car free day. Walk a friend's dog, help dig their allotment, or even get your own. You will need to address your activity level as well as your food intake.

Have realistic expectations. If you are carrying a lot of extra weight you are not going to lose it all next week, or even the week after. This is not a plan that you follow until you are slim and then abandon, with the inevitable consequences. The truth is that we need to make changes for the rest of our lives. We need to EAT LESS *and* MOVE MORE from now on.

But lets start by picking one day each week when we'll try to EAT LESS *and* MOVE MORE. It can be any day, not necessarily the same one each week. If you manage then congratulate yourself. Have a reward, but try to think of one that isn't chocolate! If it doesn't happen try again another day or next week. Ignore the times it doesn't happen and feel good about the times it does. Focus on one day at a time. Today I'm going to EAT LESS *and* MOVE MORE.

This is not a quick fix. This is gradual change that will make a difference in the long term. Start with one day a week and increase that to two days when you feel ready. Stay with this until you are ready to move up to three days, and so on up to five days a week. You can stick at any number you want to, and have days off whenever you like. Remember to do both things; EAT LESS *and* MOVE MORE.

Work through this book looking for clues to help you break out of the diet binge cycle. You may like to finish the book before you make a start.

16

Have you heard yourself say?

I haven't moved off the chair for 20 years
What a great place to start. Think of something that will prompt you such as your favourite soap starting or the adverts coming on. When that happens pick up the paper or a magazine and turn the pages. Or brush your hair. When a quiz show comes on point to the person you think will answer each question. If answering quiz questions is not your thing then think of the most unlikely answer you can and have a good laugh about it.

I cannot afford to join the gym
Going to the gym is not part of the Simplest Diet Ever. Moving more is. Choose something that suits your budget, personality and fitness level. Walking is a very good option for many people. You could combine it with window shopping, exercising the dog, or exploring a new place. You could listen to music while you walk, or even learn another language. Remember to consider your personal safety at all times.

I like music but I don't play an instrument
Thinking of something you like can set you on the right track for finding ways to move more. Put on some music, let your feet tap to the rhythm, conduct the orchestra, play an air guitar, or boogie. Why not write a song or have lessons on an instrument? Organise a party of friends to go to a musical, or be a volunteer usher at a concert venue.

I'm much too busy to find time to exercise
You are looking for opportunities to move more. It does not have to be in the form of something traditionally labelled as exercise. If you want to find an excuse you will, but if you really want to follow the Simplest Diet Ever there will be ways to fit moving more into your busy day. Try marching on the spot while the kettle is boiling or when you clean your teeth.

I live alone and don't know anyone

There are positives even in this lonely situation. There is no one else to sabotage your diet, laugh when you dance around to the advert jingles, or complain when you are building a model or jigsaw on the dining room table. Once you start to get your weight under control you will feel better about yourself and more able to offer friendship.

I already go to lots of groups

That's great. Think through the different ones considering which involve activity rather than just sitting. You are a joiner so join a group that does something active, darts, line dancing, patchwork, painting, or aerobics. If you are overweight but already do a lot of exercise look for ways of increasing the frequency, speed or length of sessions. You may need to change to something that is more vigorous or one that uses different parts of the body. Exercising in water is great for large people.

I sit down all day at work

Look for opportunities to move. You could move your feet and legs about under the desk. Offer to go and make the coffee or deliver something by using the stairs rather than the lift. Use your meal breaks to go for a walk or a swim. Think about your journey to and from work. Could you make that more active?

I can't go to a class, I'm a single parent

You don't need to go to a class. You are looking for ways to move more during your normal everyday activity. Children are active so join in with them. Instead of watching them play, play with them. Teach them how to skip, or knit. Go for a bike ride together, or a picnic. See how many different leaves you can collect and make a collage with them, or use them as stepping-stones.

Chapter 2

Eat your words

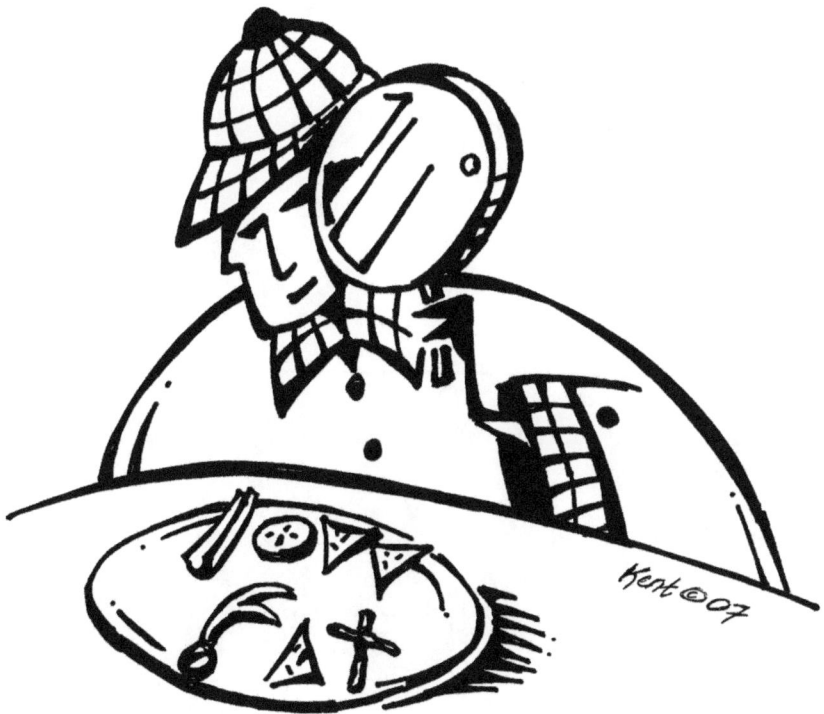

Diet jargon busted

Banks know how to change currency. You can pay into your account money from different countries and the bank knows how to change it all to the money that you use. You can pay into your body all sorts of different foods and the body knows how to change them so that they are usable.

The currency that the body uses is called calories. When you eat picture a person called Cal at the counter of your bank taking it all from you and changing it into useable currency. Your bank can pay all your bills like, heating, electric and gas, which keep your home going. Cal pays all the bills that keep your body going, by spending calories.

Calorie is from the Latin word for heat. You may have heard the expression 'to burn calories'. It is a measurement of energy, how much heat it takes to alter the temperature of a particular amount of water. So we use it to measure how much energy we get from our food.

When we eat it's like building a house with bricks and mortar and roof tiles. The bricks are made of proteins, picture cubes of cheese or meat, piles of beans, chunks of egg and fish. These are held together with mortar made of fat. Picture mixing butter or lard with vegetable oil to get the right thickness of mix to spread on the bricks.

The roof tiles are made of slices of bread and cake, neatly placed cookies and sheets of lasagne. There are slices of potato and banana, next to layers of mango and pineapple. The whole roof and the marshmallow chimney pots are liberally dusted with icing sugar until they glisten. The delivery note says carbohydrates, but the body actually sees them all as sugars.

What an amazing thing the body is; it can take all these food materials and build and grow and mend itself. Of course some individual food items contribute to the supply of more than one type of building material. Weight for weight we can build twice as much with the mortar compared with either the bricks or tiles. Fats have more than twice the calories that the same weight of sugars or proteins have. They are calorie rich.

We need supplies to keep coming in because they are being used all the time. When the order clerk sees that stocks are getting low he puts in a request for more to be delivered. In through the front door come the roof tiles, the bricks and the mortar. Sometimes it's a mixed order and sometimes it's mainly one type of material. The order is sorted and put into the kitchen cupboards. If the order is particularly large some is stored in the cupboard under the stairs.

Some order clerks get a real high when they watch the glistening roof tiles coming through the door. They just can't get enough of that feeling, never mind if the cupboard is already full, they just have to keep ordering and ordering. Some clerks like to watch the bricks coming in, they are so satisfying to stack up, so neat and tidy. Others find the mortar irresistible, it's so squishy and tactile, and they have to have more and more and more.

Cupboards are full to overflowing; even when things are being used up the replacements are there waiting. Stocks begin to build up in other places in the house. There's a pile of bricks in the hall waiting for space in the cupboard under the stairs. Roof tiles are piled in the dining room. They are pleasant colours but begin to get in the way. Mortar has wriggled under the sofa and behind the skirting boards.

The clerk just keeps right on ordering and the house starts to bulge at the seams. Build an extension, yes that's a good plan. We can grind all the extra bricks and tiles down and make it into mortar, it'll be easier to store it that way. Soon the extension is full and we have to build another. We take up the floorboards and the fat flows down into the cellar and fills that up too.

The order clerk tried to be controlled but he was enticed by special offers and the beautiful sight of the glistening tiles coming through the door. However much he wanted to, he just couldn't reduce the orders.

We are just like this house. Growing and growing even when we don't want to. Sometimes it's like we are fighting with ourselves. There is a conflict going on inside us. So we may need our hearts soothed and our spirits encouraged before we tackle food issues.

How do I choose the right diet?

You can opt to eat less of your normal meals.
You do not need to follow a set plan.

First be realistic about what you can manage. The idea is to succeed, not to set yourself up for a fall. Remember that you can start by making a change just one day a week, unless you chose to go to a slimming club where you will be expected to follow a daily plan. Think about how much control you have over what you eat.

If you are responsible for feeding others, think about whether or not they also need to make changes. This is a delicate area and may need to be negotiated. Don't assume everyone will want to join you, or that everyone will be helpful and encouraging. Some people may not be ready or willing to give it a go. Some will be determined to make you trip up. Be careful who you tell and who you involve. This is about you getting sorted. Others may follow when they see you succeed.

See which description, or sentence, seems to fit your personality and situation the nearest. Take up the suggestions that you feel will help you, and that are viable for you.

Many of us are very experienced failures when it comes to diets. We have those experiences and possibly other emotional baggage to sort out. Remember that we are not just focusing on our physical bodies. In later chapters we will be exploring the need to soothe our hearts, awaken our spirituality, and alter our thinking patterns as we tackle our baggage. If it all feels too threatening to contemplate, please wait until you have read the rest of the book before deciding how to change your eating.

Others prepare all of my meals.
I don't want to change what I eat.
I always end up focusing on food and eating more.
Carry on eating what you normally eat, but eat less of it.
Drink lots of water.
Focus on looking for opportunities to move more.

I don't want to have to weigh or measure anything.
I could manage small changes but nothing major.
I'm willing to try changes one day a week.
Small changes will make a difference.

Ten tips for small changes
1. Cut food up smaller and use smaller plates.
2. Only put spread on one piece of bread for each sandwich.
3. Drink plenty of water before and during meals.
4. Fill up on vegetables.
5. Bake or grill rather than fry.
6. Enjoy the taste of the food when it's in your mouth.
7. Trim the fat off meat.
8. Put the cutlery down occasionally between mouthfuls.
9. Reduce the number of times you have fast food.
10. Eat fruit or vegetables for snacks.

I want someone to prepare my meals for me.

There are plenty of tasty ready prepared, sometimes pre-cooked, meals available in every supermarket. All the counting, weighing and measuring has been done for you. You must just decide what criteria you are going to use to help you choose wisely, perhaps meals that are no more than 3% fat or within a particular calorie range. The portions will probably not be as big as you are used to, but eating less is the simplest diet ever.

There are meal replacement drinks on the market and they too have the nutritional input all sorted for you. There are companies that will arrange your complete diet and deliver all the meal replacements to you. Some people find using meal replacement drinks really helpful. My only caution would be that, unless you plan to use these drinks for the rest of your life, at some point you will have to switch back to solid food and learn to eat less of it

I'm willing to consider following a set diet plan.
I prepare my own meals.
I want to understand how diet plans work.
Tell me what to do and I'll give it a try.

If a diet works it's because it has helped you eat less, so that you have paid in less calories. Some plans encourage or include an exercise programme and that's getting the body to spend more calories by using up energy. Whatever the label, packaging, presentation, scientific proof or marvellous new discovery, they all work because you take in less calories.

They cause you to control your intake of one or more of the basic three food groups, that's protein bricks or sugar tiles or fatty mortar. We have gone through a craze of calorie controlled and then low fat diets. The latest fashion is to select particular types of sugars that satisfy the body for longer. That certainly makes a lot of sense.

There are books, magazines, web sites and often clubs which will help you restrict your intake of some foods, and advise you about menus and recipes. Remember that if you have tried one particular diet plan several times before, now is a good time to change to something else.

Diets explained

Low calorie diets
These recommend the total number of calories you should consume in a day. You can be free to get to that total in any way you like, or to follow a diet plan that gives lists of meals and snacks to choose from. Ready prepared meals fit well here.

Low fat diets
Fats are calorie rich so you can significantly reduce your calorie intake by controlling your fat intake. Most dairy products like cheese, milk, butter, and yoghurt, are available in lower fat versions including some that are almost fat free. Look out for fat free salad dressings and reduced fat sauces. Again ready meals are useful here, particularly the ones that are 3% fat or less.

Fats fall into two main groups, those that are solid when you go to use them, and those that are liquid. The solid ones, such as butter, are called saturated and have a nasty habit of leaving fatty deposits in the blood vessels. That's what the Doctor is checking for if you have a cholesterol test. Think Solid; Saturate; Sludge! It's healthier to have the group of fats that are liquid e.g. Olive oil or vegetable oil. Also avoid products with hydrogenated fat. You are looking out for vegetable rather than animal fats. It's healthier still to eat less fat altogether.

Ten tips for eating less fat
1. Bake or grill instead of frying.
2. Use oven instead of fried chips. Straight cut rather than crinkle cut.

26

3. Substitute quark, a very low fat cheese, for butter on bread and baked potatoes.
4. Try fat free fromage frais in place of cream.
5. Have less fast food.
6. When roasting, spray on the oil rather than pouring it on.
7. Remove visible fat and skin from meat and poultry.
8. Drain off the fat before making gravy.
9. Snack on fruit and vegetables.
10. Reduce the amount of cheese you eat.

Low protein diets

These restrict the amount of meats, poultry, fish, cheese, nuts and other foods that contain protein. You could choose to eat smaller servings of these foods, or follow a plan that will instruct you about the weight and portion sizes. Remember that many individual food items are made up of more than one of the food groups, so don't be surprised to see them crop up in several of the diets. Dairy products like milk and cheese are examples.

We often add fats or oils when we eat proteins. We fry them, coat them in oil, or have a creamy sauce. When we eat less proteins we also eat less of the fats that we usually have with them, which further reduces our calorie intake.

Tips for a low protein diet
1. Slice thinner and dice smaller so that a small portion looks plentiful.
2. Increase vegetables and tomato in meat sauces.
3. Nibble fruit rather than cheese.
4. Barbecue vegetable kebabs to have with smaller meat or fish portions.
5. Plan meals around pasta, potato or rice.
6. Feature a vegetable. Fill a pepper, tomato or mushroom.
7. Have big colourful mixed salads with just a little protein.
8. Careful with peanut snacks and peanut butter.
9. Take a burger or steak one size down from your usual order.
10. Move away from having full English breakfasts.

Low carbohydrate diets

These restrict your intake of cereals, flour, bread, cakes, biscuits, cookies, pasta, rice, potatoes, pastry, sugar, and foods with high sugar content. Again you could simply opt to eat less of these, or go for a diet plan that will tell you suitable portion sizes, menus, and recipes.

Often low carbohydrate diet plans have a low fat element combined with them. Strict vegetarians may not find a low carbohydrate plan suitable as they have less protein options.

Tips for a low carbohydrate diet.
1. Plan your meals around protein foods like meat, fish, quorn, or eggs.
2. Have the meat and veg part of a full English breakfast. Remember to grill not fry.
3. Barbecues are ideal. Have plenty of different meats or fish for variety.
4. Roast onions, leeks and carrots to have with a joint of meat.
5. Reduce your portions of potato, parsnips, peas and sweet corn.
6. Eat plenty of other vegetables and salads.
7. Add carrot and swede before mashing potatoes.
8. Eat out at the Carvery or Steak houses.
9. Snack on fish sticks, prawns, and raw vegetables.
10. Drink more water and less sugared drinks, alcohol, pop and fruit juice.

Many of our usual everyday snacks and packed lunches are carbohydrate rich. As are the goodies we have when friends come over for coffee. So we will need to be creative in finding alternatives. Instead of coffee and cake, why not have coffee with dessert and make a colourful fruit salad to have with yoghurt.

28

Glycaemic index

Some carbohydrates are in a form that the body can very quickly extract the sugar from. However others come with lots of packaging that the digestive process takes time to remove before the sugar can be extracted. The time taken also varies depending on which other foods are eaten at the same meal, as some further hamper the process of sugar extraction.

By selecting to eat carbohydrates that have the sugars well wrapped up you will feel satisfied for longer. When we eat carbs that have readily available sugars we get a sugar rush and then a low, where upon we feel like we need to eat again. Each food is given an index number relating to how quickly the body gets the sugar into the blood stream. The higher the number the quicker the body gets the sugar. Think of it as miles per hour. This speed is reduced when travelling with certain other vehicles. Although this diet is based around eating carbohydrates you will end up eating less of them because you won't be hungry so often.

Tips for the glycaemic index (G.I.) diet.
1. Plan your meals around low G.I. carbs and veg.
2. Use artificial sweeteners instead of sugar.
3. Have low calorie drinks or water.
4. Fibre is your friend. Add bran to any meal you can.
5. Restrict low G.I. foods that are high in fat content.
6. Eat more porridge.
7. Use wholemeal bread and pasta rather than white.
8. The less processed the better.
9. Have plenty of fruit and vegetables.
10. Many low G.I. foods make great soup.

Don't be put off by these two carbohydrate pathways. If you want to try one just be clear which one you want to follow and stick with it. Remember that you can choose to make changes on just one day a week to start with. And you can choose not to be concerned about food groups or diet plans at all, but simply eat less of the things you normally eat.

DRINKS

As well as adjusting your eating, you can also make a difference by changing your drinking habits. Do this gradually, and experiment until you find changes that suit you. Again start with one day a week. You are aiming to reduce the calories you consume in liquid form. Have a look at the labels on your drinks, or look up the values, to get an overall view of how they add up.

When our blood sugar level rises and then drops we start to feel hungry. The sugar/carbohydrate in our drinks contributes to this rise and fall, just as it does with our food intake. It will help us to EAT LESS if we trigger the feeling of hunger as little as possible. We can do this by reducing the number of sweet drinks we have and by selecting drinks that have no, or only low, sugar content.

Some people have a much more acute sense of taste than others do. Some of us are able to switch to low calorie versions of a drink without a problem about the taste, whilst others can't. If you can't find acceptable low calorie drinks then make a straight swap on some occasions between your sweet drink and water.

WATER

Increase your intake of water. It's calorie free, great for hydration, and it's filling. Try a glass before meals and one during. Use big glasses for water.

MILK

The lower the fat content in the milk the lower the calories. So a switch to skimmed or semi-skimmed milk will save you calories. You don't necessarily have to use the same type of milk all the time. If you prefer full cream on your cereal but can manage with skimmed or semi-skimmed in drinks then make that change. Every little helps.

MILKSHAKE

The calorie values of milkshakes differ enormously depending on the type of milk used and what has been added for flavour and texture. Most often lots of sugar or a syrup mixture and maybe cream or ice cream. I'm afraid that no milkshakes are low in calories. Just one of those wonderful large size shakes from fast food outlets can contain nearly all the calories you need in a whole day!

If you drink lots of milkshake then you have hit upon the very thing to cut down on in order to help you lose weight. A glass of milk alone is better than a milkshake.

Some of us have successfully persuaded ourselves that since milk is good for us then milkshakes must be even better. We mix and match that thought with the fact that there are milkshakes, all be it intended as meal replacements, on some diets. Thus we come up with the idea that they are an excellent healthy option. We are so easily deceived when it suits us!

How are we going to give them up without feeling deprived and ending up craving them even more? Instead of telling yourself you can't have them, try telling yourself that you can have them whenever you like, provided it's your birthday!

CAFFEINE

Drinks like tea, coffee and cola contain it. Some of the drinks that are intended to boost energy levels and keep you awake have high caffeine content. It is also found in some medicines. Check out the labels. Caffeine causes a sudden rise in blood sugar levels, just as eating or drinking sugar does. That's why we like it! After the rise comes the fall. So it also triggers our hunger. Having decaffeinated drinks helps to keep the blood sugar level more even so we feel satisfied for longer. Consider making the switch for all, or some, of your drinks.

FIZZY POP

Ordinary pop is packed with sugar. Go for the low calorie versions whenever possible. A recent study found that large people drink far more of all types of pop, including low calorie ones, than smaller people. If we want to join the smaller people perhaps we should drink less pop too.

FRUIT JUICES AND SMOOTHIES

Fruit is an important part of our diet and we should try to have it regularly. When we eat raw fruit it takes the body time to break it down. When we liquidise fruit, the breaking down happens in the machine, before we drink it, so it is much more quickly digested. The inevitable result is that the natural sugars cause a quicker rise in blood sugar. Then comes the drop, and then the hunger.

It takes several fruits to make enough for a glass of juice. So the juice is much higher in calories than one piece of fruit. Be careful not to be tempted to down a large carton. To save calories use a smaller glass and consider diluting juices with water. You can add low fat yoghurt to smoothies to slow down the sugar rush.

MEAL REPLACEMENT DRINKS

Don't be tempted to use them as a snack or just as a drink. Don't confuse these with 'diet drinks'. They are high in calories, and will sabotage your efforts unless used instead of a meal.

ALCOHOL

Newspapers regularly publish articles boasting of the health value of this or that type of alcohol, only to contradict it later. You can probably find something in writing to justify anything you want to drink. If you like to have alcohol try and keep it to a small amount. A large intake is poisonous to the body and harmful. If your eating is in excess, then your drinking may be as well. Now is the time to take back control of both. Reducing your alcohol intake will reduce your calories too.

Quick quiz

Just answer YES or NO and total up each column

Do you enjoy eating	YES	NO
Lettuce		
Grapefruit		
Chicken		
Yoghurt		
Sago pudding		
Cabbage soup		
Lentils		
Apples		
Bread		
Tomato Soup		
Gravy		
Scrambled eggs		
Chocolate		
Prawns		
Melon		
Cheese		
Pork chops		
Bananas		
Cake		
Carrots		
Prunes		

	YES	NO
Total		

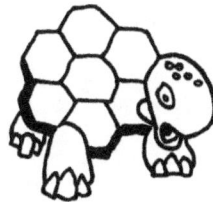

Score 0 - 21
It doesn't matter how many YES or NO you put!
All the things you don't like you don't have to eat.
All the things you do like you can have.

If you choose the simplest diet possible all you have to do is EAT LESS of what you normally eat *and* MOVE MORE. If you are eating the things you like now, carry on eating them. If you choose to follow a diet plan then you are buying into some restrictions about the selection of food you eat as well as portion sizes. Consider your personal likes and dislikes when you think about how you are going to eat less. Don't torture yourself with a lettuce diet if you don't like lettuce.

We would all like a quick fix diet. We would like to wake up in the morning and be slim, healthy, married to a millionaire............need I go on? There is a way to be strong and beautiful, and we will come onto that later. For now the best we can do is wake up in the morning and say 'Today I will eat less and move more'.

Those who have dieted before will be familiar with charts that show ideal weight for your height, or the relationship between the two, called the Body Mass Index (B.M.I.). If you find it helpful to know these figures then go ahead and look that up. But if targets and weight loss expectations add to your distress, and send you running to the fridge, don't look them up at all.

You know if you are too fat, and you know if you want to do something about it. If you do, then you are reading the right book. If you think you are fat but your family and friends say you are not, then go and talk to the Doctor and let him advise you.

Chapter 3

Bodies behaving badly

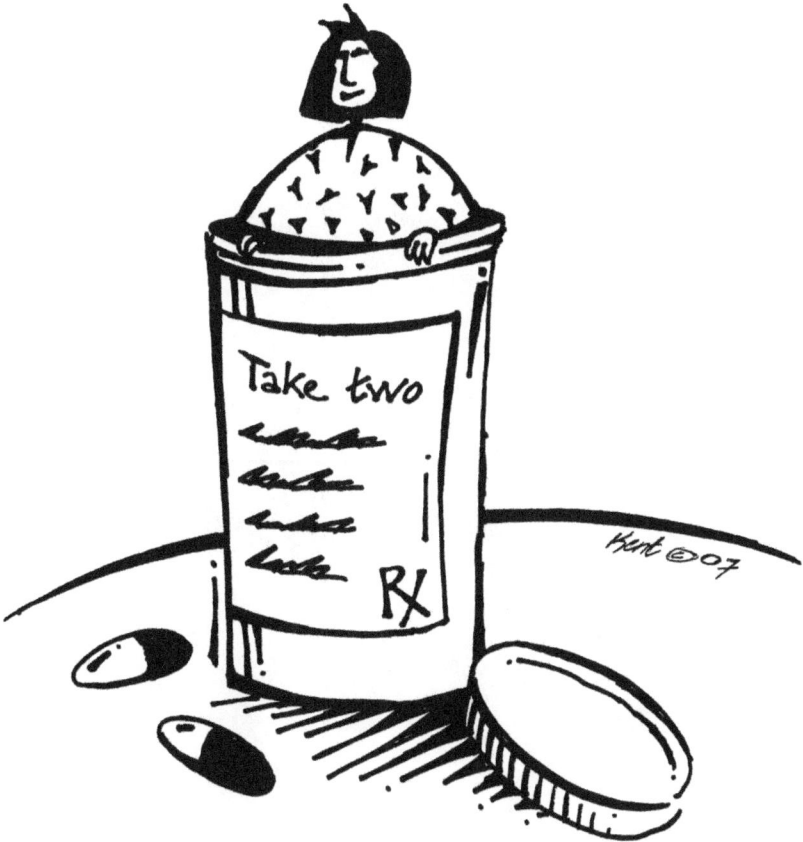

Medical conditions and weight gain

Every day you get the bus to work. You have a routine, but you are so used to it that it just comes naturally. You have a time you get up, do what you have to do, and leave the house in time to get to the bus stop. Meanwhile the bus has set off from the depot and is making it's way to you. Round about the same time each morning it comes along and you get on.

However one day you don't get on that bus. Perhaps you pressed the snooze button on the alarm clock. Maybe the battery ran out all together. Or perhaps you have been setting it one minute later everyday and now you are running late. You were held up. The phone went, the toast burnt setting off the fire alarm, the cat is petrified and was sick over your coat. The bus came and left without you.

Another day, when you are at the bus stop on time, the bus doesn't come. You may never know why. Maybe the driver was sick, or the depot vandalised. The bus got a puncture, or was held up by an accident or roadworks. Endless possibilities. Your usual routine didn't happen that morning. You and the bus didn't meet.

Our bodies routines and systems have to coincide, one affecting the other. Most of the time this just happens. We don't have to tell our body that tea or coffee is on the way, nor advise it on how to absorb it. When we are running for the bus, and need extra energy, the body knows it needs to burn calories.

The body has a clock. It has a rhythm like a pendulum swinging, which keeps the processes going on schedule.

Eating, digesting, energy distribution, waste disposal, growth and development. This is our metabolism

The speed at which our metabolism works is adjusted by some of our glands. For instance, the thyroid gland can become over active, then all the body processes will work too quickly, using up vast amounts of energy and causing the fat stores to be raided for everyday use.

UNDER ACTIVE THYROID
If the thyroid gland sets the levels too low, because it is not working properly, then everything slows down, less energy is used and the fat stores continue to build up. Excess fluid is held in the cells causing swelling, often of the face, tongue, and ankles. Along with weight gain and swelling other symptoms include a slowing down of the thought process, lethargy, depression, dry skin, hoarse voice, and hair loss, particularly the outer part of the eye brows. This condition usually comes on slowly, although you can be born with it. It is more common in woman than men, and also more common in people with Down's Syndrome.

POLYCYSTIC OVARY DISEASE
Another medical condition that causes women to gain weight is Polycystic Ovary disease. Other symptoms include period problems, fertility problems and excess body and facial hair.

There are also other conditions that affect weight. If you have a medical condition that causes weight gain then you are faced with an added challenge when trying to lose weight. It is harder, but not impossible. EAT LESS *and* MOVE MORE is an ideal plan for you. You will find controlling your carbohydrate intake particularly helpful, so consider the Glycaemic Index plan.

You may have noticed that the Simplest Diet Ever logo is a tortoise. Slow and steady gets there in the end. Be glad about each small step in the right direction.

Alongside your medical condition there may be other life issues contributing to your chaotic eating. Having a medical condition can be a reason and an excuse for over eating.

A healthy body can tell you when it is hungry and needs food. It can also tell us when we have had enough, and when we have overdone it!

PRADA-WILLI SYNDROME
Unfortunately this cycle of communication can fail. For instance, those with Prada-Willi Syndrome have an insatiable hunger all the time. If you have this syndrome then you face an incredible challenge, but it's not impossible. If you EAT LESS *and* MOVE MORE you will increase your life quality and expectancy. You will have to be prepared to tolerate feeling hungry. Getting involved in activities that take place where food isn't available will really help.

This condition is extremely rare. Many of us think we feel hungry all the time, but we haven't really got a problem with our body chemistry. Ours is more an emotional hunger and comfort eating.

HEALTH PROBLEMS WHICH PREVENT ACTIVITY
As well as medical conditions that cause direct weight gain, there are others where weight gain can occur because less activity is possible. Our eating may stay the same, but we burn up fewer calories because we move less, resulting in weight gain.

This can occur if we are less active for a long period with a complicated pregnancy, following an accident, or due to a long-term condition. Also with illnesses such as depression, chronic fatigue (M.E.), and post viral syndrome, because the normal range of everyday activities cannot continue.

Of course being overweight can itself lead us to be less active, which in turn leads us to put on more weight; a viscous circle that has to be broken. Your ability to exercise will increase as you exercise.

The balance can be redressed if you EAT LESS *and* MOVE MORE. Discuss the best way to do this with the health professionals who are caring for you. If not all of you can move then move the bits that can. If you are in the recovery stage of a condition that causes fatigue try increasing your activity level by just one or two footsteps each day.

DEPRESSION
Walking is very beneficial for anyone with depression. Not only will it help you keep your weight under control, but it also causes the body to produce happy hormone (Serotonin) that will help to lift your mood. Start with a regular short walk and increase gradually.

Part way through the walk stop somewhere you can sit for a while, perhaps a park or a church. Give yourself this time to think about some of the things on you mind. People with depression often don't sleep very well, perhaps getting off to sleep ok but waking in the early hours with thoughts going round and round. If you allow space in the day to process some of your thoughts, such as a break part way through a walk, you may find that you can sleep better.

You need to explore the life issues that are causing your depression as well as the over eating. They may be one and the same. The thing that finally tipped you over into depression may not be the only, or even the main, issue for you, just the final straw. Look out in particular for past situations where you need to accept, and work through, your anger.

Chapter five has more about dealing with life issues, and also altering the way you think.

40

MEDICATION
Medications, such as steroids, the contraceptive pill and HRT, can cause weight gain. So can giving up smoking, as smoking suppresses the appetite. The Simplest Diet Ever is suitable in all these cases.

Diabetics, who want to lose weight and increase exercise, should be aware that the amount of insulin required to maintain a normal blood sugar level may need to be reduced. People who take medication for conditions such as under active thyroid, asthma, or high cholesterol, may also find that their dose can be reduced as they lose weight

Remember that it is advisable to visit your Doctor if you have a medical condition, take medication, or have not exercised recently. Continue taking your normal medication unless the Doctor makes a change.

WEIGHT GAIN AFFECTS OUR HEALTH
There are medical conditions that cause us to gain weight or be less active. However there are far more medical problems caused due to weight gain.

There is an increased risk of:

> High blood pressure
> Heart attacks
> Strokes
> Breathing problems
> Joint problems
> Diabetes type 2
> Blood clots
> Mobility problems
> Fertility problems
> Asthma
> Cancer
> ....to name just a few

These risks increase as the weight increases.

A study in the USA found that severely obese young men were 12 times more likely to die than their lighter friends. Twelve times!

Is that a risk worth taking?

By being overweight we are actually causing harm to ourselves. But by losing just a tenth (10%) of our body weight we will considerably reduce the risks.

The time to act is now. Before it's too late.

Present health concerns
Action I want to take

Chapter 4

One size fits all

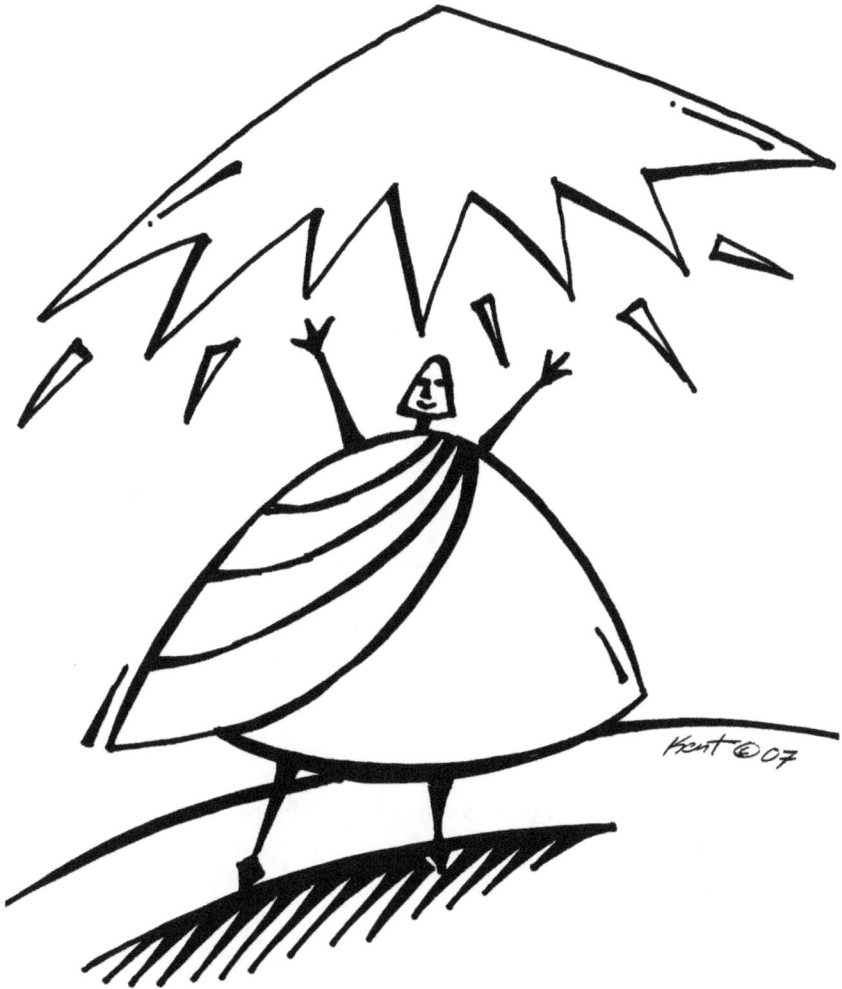

Due to wonderful medical advances, doctors are sometimes able to restart the hearts of people who would otherwise die. Television hospital dramas are popular viewing. You may be able to picture a resuscitation room and hear 'stand clear' before the paddles are put on the casualty's chest.

When this occurs in reality the patient is briefly dead. The heart has stopped beating but then life is restarted. These people can often describe what happened to them during that brief death experience. The similarities in these accounts are fascinating.

Most describe being able to look at their own body as they float away from it. There is always some kind of tunnel with a light at the end. When their heart is restarted they experience going back into their body. How can this be a coincidence?

If you have been unsure about any sort of life after death, then these plentiful accounts will be of significance to you. How could they see anything, tunnels and light, after death unless part of them, their spirit, was still alive?

What has this got to do with a diet? We are approaching our food issues from a holistic point of view, by looking at our whole being, body, mind, heart, and spirit. When people lose weight, only concentrating on their body, four out of five will put the weight back on again. If we are going to be consistent with our weight loss we need to look at the bigger picture. You need to see yourself as a whole person.

We know that life on this earth is temporary. Those who have briefly experience death, report that it is not the end. If we go on living after our life here on earth, do we have any say about it? Does anything that we do here on earth, or any of the choices that we make, affect where we go when we die? Who is in control of that? There is no threat in exploring faith. There might even be great gain in awakening our spirituality.

God didn't have anybody quite like you, so he made you. He thinks you're amazing. The Bible says He knows all about you, and he still thinks you're amazing. He loves you, and will never take that love away, even if you never lose a pound! In fact he wants you to be part of his family. He gives you an invitation to belong to him. This offer is 'one size fits all'.

God invites us to go on from here to live with him in heaven forever. We don't have a full understanding of what it will be like but the Bible does tell us that we get a new body. This body will be strong, healthy, and beautiful. There will be no pain, no tears, no sickness.

Death is a difficult subject for us to think about. We would rather not think about it. Yet, if there are options about what happens next don't we owe it to ourselves to investigate? By carrying too much weight we are likely to get there sooner than our contemporaries. All the more reason to think about it now!

God's word, the Bible, also tells us about our behaviour. It says we do the things we don't want to do, and we don't do the things we should. God knows how hard we find it to EAT LESS *and* MOVE MORE. He knows when we sit down to read a slimming magazine and eat our way through a chocolate bar or two at the same time. He is not in the least surprised that we mess up. His love is unconditional.

God isn't surprised about our food issues. God created people. We are different from animals because we have the unique ability to relate to God. God calls and we can answer. Responding to God affects our life now and what happens when our life on earth comes to an end. When God created the first man and woman he gave them a beautiful garden to enjoy. Even in that perfect setting they were tempted over food and they blew it.

Like Adam and Eve we mess up. We hurt people and we get hurt. Whilst not liking all we do, God still loves us, and wants us to get to know him. He can also separate us from our wrong behaviour in another sense. He promises to completely forgive all our wrong doing if we ask him to. Nothing we have done will surprise him because he already knows it all.

God loves us so much that he sent Jesus, his only son, to the rescue. What an amazing thing to do. In my work as a children's nurse I've seen the parents distress when their child is suffering. God, as a Father, sent his son to suffer and die. We are clearly the guilty ones, but Jesus took the punishment so that we can be forgiven.

We need to change from going our own way to going God's way. Jesus died for us so our wrongdoing can be forgiven. We can accept the offer of being in his family and have a place in Heaven. We can invite Jesus into our lives, ask for forgiveness, and invite the Holy Spirit to fill us. Jesus is still saying 'Come follow me', just as he did to the fisherman two thousand years ago. God beckons, draws us, calls us.

The Holy Spirit, God's presence in those who have found faith through Jesus, is described as a counsellor and a comforter. As we come to look at our hearts, to see if they need soothing, we may be in need of comfort and counsel.

When we awaken our understanding of ourselves as spiritual beings our life can take on a whole new direction and purpose. The Bible is God's handbook for living. Mark's Gospel is a good place to start. It's near the beginning of the second section called The New Testament.

Prayer is having a conversation with God, both talking and listening. Why not give it a try?

God, if you are there, please reveal yourself to me. Help me to understand how much you love me.

Chapter 5

Busy getting nowhere

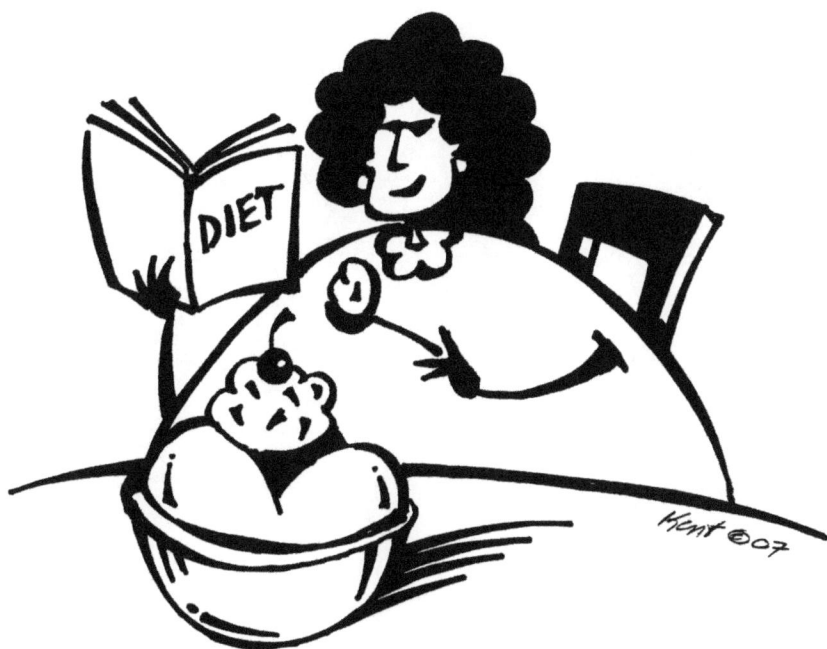

You may attribute the blame for the way you eat to someone else. Certainly there are families where everyone is eating portions that are too large, and that becomes the norm. Food is enjoyable, available, and tied into celebration, comfort, reward, and our desire to be good providers. We need to move past blame to action, and we have to take action for ourselves.

There are many recognised reasons for why we overeat. Some people say it is just a habit. But we can learn to break habits. So why are we still fat? Why do we lose weight only to put it all back on, and sometimes more? Our weight goes up and down like a yo-yo. If we manage to control what we eat for a period of time it doesn't seem to help with our long-term lifestyle issues. Perhaps there is more to it than habit.

Overeating can be an addiction. We can feel powerless to control it. Food controls us and we binge. There is some sort of relief gained by binge eating. Unlike other addictions we can't plan to give up totally. We need to eat and drink to stay alive. So we need to get to a place where we are free from the need to overeat.

Overeating is an emotional crutch. Many people can relate to the concept of comfort eating. But less of us are aware that it can be a response to unresolved life issues. We eat to mask our feelings. We push our feelings inside and cover them with food. We overeat because we are sad, and then we're sad because we've eaten!

People respond very differently to the same situation. How we connect to, and express, our emotions is linked to our culture, family life, individual personality, and the amount of previous emotional events that we have dealt with. We are affected by the inherited personality traits in our genes, and by the way we have been bought up.

We also have an automatic protective mechanism that we may not be aware of. This can come into play when we have been hurt, without us realising it has been triggered. For example, people who have been deeply hurt by a failed relationship, and those who have been sexually abused, may put on weight so that they are less attractive, thus less likely to be hurt again. It isn't a conscious action, it's the automatic protective system at work. Imagine the conflict in such a person when they try to lose weight. Part of them is saying it's safer to stay big and part of them wants to be smaller. Some resolution needs to happen before the person is free to deal with their weight problem.

With relationship break-ups, we see food becoming a weapon used by separated parents and shared care children. Parents desperate to maintain popularity can be inadvertently tempted to overindulge the child as a way of expressing their love. Children soon pick up on the rewarding possibility of manipulating the situation so that each parent feels the need to outdo the other with trips to fast food outlets and sweet treats. Of course this can happen in any family, not just those with relationship problems.

Food can be really quite powerful. Even a toddler can learn to create havoc for their parents by refusing to eat. Our relationship with food goes far beyond the need to provide our body with nourishment. Changing our relationship to food will not come easy. We might be attending a slimming club, or reading every new diet book that comes out. But the act of attending or reading doesn't necessarily bring about any change in our eating.

We can be seemingly putting great effort into dieting but we are in fact busy getting nowhere. It won't do just to look at our body when we want to lose weight. We must grasp that there is more going on in us that can affect our eating. Few of us can successfully deal with our eating issues until we have dealt with our life issues. That's why we need to be looking at our hearts, minds and spirits as well as our bodies.

We need to spring clean our emotional baggage. Some baggage will be easy to sort out, and other baggage will cling as if it's attached with those stretchy octopus bungees that we use to hold luggage on the car roof. It may take time to prise the elasticated hooks off one by one. Sometimes we have been carrying baggage for so long it has become an integral part of who we are.

Every life has a smattering of emotional events which cause a response, or reaction, and eventually some sort of resolution in that we learn to live with them. You may have heard of the grief process. In this situation the event is a death. The response may be any combination and order of emotions from anger, disbelief, sadness, regret, relief, despair, crying, and constantly retelling the story, until you adjust and learn to live without the person. It can be a very long and painful process.

It may be that you have been bereaved but never had the opportunity to express these emotions. Some cultures expect people to express grief in an open way and other cultures discourage any display of emotions. What happens to emotions that we can't express? Some of us pop them into our baggage and we eat to cover them up.

Sometimes we don't connect our turmoil of feelings with the death. This can particularly happen with children who haven't been warned that they might feel grief. It can also happen with an adult two years, or even ten years, after the event at which point they don't connect the loss to the resurgence of strong emotions.

Also one death can open the floodgates of emotion from a previous bereavement, piling pain on pain. We expect people to be upset after a death. However we can experience similar emotions after all sorts of 'loss or change' events, and may be covering those up with food too.

Emotional pain is hard to describe. It's not a visible wound that people can see and respond to. Some people feel the need to have something that actually causes physical pain to somehow make sense of having inner pain. They may harm themselves by cutting or burning. We cause ourselves harm by overeating.

We do not always have a smooth path on to resolution after an emotional event. Sometimes we get stuck in the shadow of the event and continue our destructive behaviour pattern such as binge eating, cutting, drinking, drug taking, or some other form of self-harm. We are using this behaviour as a way of coping.

Think through the events in your life and the way you have responded. You may need help with this. Does anything still have an emotional charge about it? You are looking to make a connection between emotions and eating, and for situations that need some unpacking. The follow lists are just a starting point. You could tick them, link across from one to the other, or add to them from your experience.

EMOTIONAL EVENTS
Bereavements
Rejection
Adoption/fostering/ becoming an evacuee
Becoming obese
Abuse (physical, emotional, sexual, or neglect)
Misunderstanding
Disappointment
Violence
Other people's expectations
Redundancy
Crime
Trauma
Bullying
Sibling rivalry
Infertility
Loss of health
Changing school/college/job
Loss of independence
Depression
Changing location
Loss of status
Family problems
Separation
Divorce
Parental conflict
Alcoholic parent or partner
Betrayal
Regretted actions or words
Parenthood
Gender or sexuality issues
Retirement
Disfigurement
Homelessness/ becoming a refugee
Debt
Disease
Failure

RESPONSE

Anger
Disbelief
Regret
Sadness
Guilt
Fear
Crying
Feeling of emotional charge
Drug abuse
Alcohol abuse
Need to retell the story over and over
Acute loneliness
Despair
Depression
Aggression
Withdrawal
Running away
Less appetite
More appetite
Over eating
Under eating
Binge eating
Self induced vomiting
Self loathing
Craving attention
Phobias
Apportioning blame
Self harm
Problems sleeping
Anxiety
Promiscuity
Difficulty trusting people
Problems building relationships
Suicidal thoughts/actions
Changes to personal grooming
Loss of self worth/esteem
Criminal activity

We all know people who have never moved on after a distressing event and it still dominates their life years later. I am not suggesting that we ever completely get over things. But we can learn to live with them.

Over eating is usually seen as the problem. But it may be more accurate to see it as the response to a problem, situation, or life issue. Making that connection, and sorting out the baggage, is not an easy task. But it is key to successful long term weight loss. Of course our eating habits and inactive life styles have to change as well.

If someone has hurt you, and part of your response has been overeating, you are allowing them to continue to hurt you all the time you continue to overeat. Is that what you really want?

Lets find new strategies and coping skills so that we can face life without the need to overeat. Ultimately we are planning to EAT LESS *and* MOVE MORE. You can start doing that at anytime. But it is perfectly ok to check out your heart, head, and spiritual needs first. Hopefully you are beginning to see how all these things are intertwined, and how important it is to deal with our eating issues from a holistic viewpoint.

Some people have found medication and/or surgery helpful in their quest to be slimmer. These can alter the digestive tract, causing substantial weight loss, but they don't address the reasons behind the overeating in the first place. If you have used these methods to get slim don't miss out on the opportunity to look further than just the body.

When we decide to face something about ourselves that we don't like, such as our size, we can feel extremely vulnerable. If we have used food to cover over emotions we are going to be even more vulnerable if we take away that shield.

As you start to lose weight you may find that your emotions are more acute or that you are distressed about issues that you didn't realise had affected you, or thought were over long ago. Try not to be too discouraged. This is exactly the connection that I am encouraging you to look for; links between eating and feelings. By sorting out unresolved life issues you are going to be better able to make permanent changes to your eating and weight.

God loves you, and is more than willing to help you deal with the things that life throws at you. Don't misunderstand this and think that there is an option not to feel emotions, because there isn't. Emotions are part of who we are as people made in God's image. The Bible tells us that Jesus felt all sorts of emotions and it records two situations when he cried.

God is not the enemy. Emotions are not the enemy. Food is not the enemy. Sometimes it seems like we are our own enemy. We do things that really hurt ourselves in the long run for a brief moment of pleasure, or a brief opportunity to blank out the reality of life's pain.

Jesus told us to love our neighbours as ourselves. Some of our neighbours get a pretty raw deal, because we don't love ourselves much. In fact some of us don't even like ourselves. We need to find out why that is, and start to sort out the things that have contributed to our poor self-image.

We are not looking to dwell in the past but to move forward. This may require us to stretch back and unhook those bungees so that we are free to move forward. We have to move on from where we are and not from where we would like to be. We can't alter our past, but we can take control of how it affects us now.

It can be enough simply to realise that we are covering our emotions with food. But some situations need more unpacking. You may like to ask someone to pray with you, or speak to a counsellor. It is not a weakness to seek help. It is a positive decision on your pathway towards being able to EAT LESS *and* MOVE MORE.

REWIRING THE BRAIN
Our brains have well worn pathways in them. We think of a situation and our brain will run an automatic response from its experience or learnt expectations. It can be like a broken record playing the same thing again and again.

We think of doing something about our weight and our brain tells us that it's no good going on a diet because you always fail, you'll never stick to it. You always fail. Give up before you start because you're a failure. On and on and on. We have convinced ourselves that we are a failure when it comes to dealing with food.

The same can happen when we think about exercise. Our brain reminds us of all the bad experiences and thoughts we have had, how embarrassing it will be, how awful it was in the changing room at school. Everyone else will be thin, fit, gorgeous, lycra clad experts. You don't know what to say, do, or wear. Failure again!

Our own well-worn thought paths are imprinted on our brains. So our own brain doesn't even seem to be on our side! When we think about eating less and moving more our head plays us the record entitled 'you're a failure so forget it'. To get our head back on our side we need to rewrite the pathways so that it comes up with a positive response. The Bible talks about the renewing of our minds, and that's what we need. A new way of thinking, in line with the positive way God thinks about us.

We need to start actively using our brains in situations when the action is usually made without conscious thought. When you go to the cupboard to chose a mug for a cup of tea or coffee tell your brain this is a good choice, I can succeed in drinking tea from this mug. When you sit down with the drink tell your brain that it's a good choice of chair and that you can sit on it.

Retread the pathways so that your mind starts to take onboard good choices and success. When you pick up a paper or a book, tell your brain that it's a good choice, I can be successful in reading this. Give your brain positive feedback about the choices you make, even little ones.

When you have established this way of thinking, make an active choice to follow the Simplest Diet Ever. Your brain will tell you that it's a good choice and you can succeed. Which of course it is, and you can!

Chapter 6

No smalls to wash

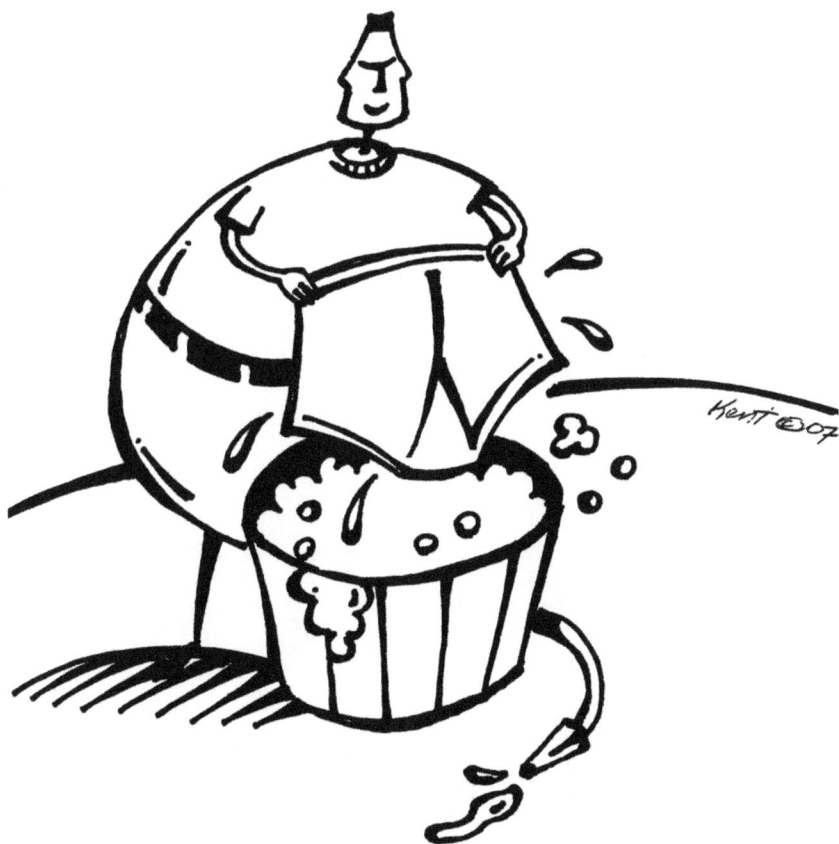

A key factor in any change process is motivation. We need to have good reasons for wanting to change. Ones that can help carry us through the tough days and keep us heading in the right direction. If you don't find the motivation to change you will carry on wearing big knickers, and never have 'smalls' to wash!

We need to be very realistic and self aware to focus on things that will keep us going. If we put too much pressure on ourselves we are in danger of reverting to comfort eating because we are stressed. Too little pressure and we will quickly give up because we are not bothered enough about being successful with the changes.

It's easy to get into a negative behaviour cycle. Once we decide that something about us is not ok, say we recognise that we are too fat and inactive, we struggle to keep ourselves together and feel sufficiently ok to do something about it. It's tempting to feel bad about having a weight problem and comfort eat even more.

We feel bad about being big. We eat more because we feel bad. We feel bad about being big. We eat more because we feel bad. The negative cycle goes on. When we focus on how we feel about ourselves we get stuck in a rut.

The value in approaching our food issues in a holistic way is that it doesn't just look at our body, or how we feel. It leads us towards the healing of our hearts. It walks us towards God and when we start to focus, not on what we feel about ourselves, but on what he thinks about us, we can get out of that rut.

God thinks you are loveable, unique, precious, forgivable, and worth dying for. Rebuild your self-esteem around God's view of you.

Think through achievements you have made in the past. Try and work out what helped you to be successful. You are looking to gain an understanding of what motivates you so that you can apply it to these new challenges of eating less and moving more. Motivation may have come from within you, from an outside source, or both.

When we were children we achieved some things because a parent, carer, or teacher helped us. That may have included correcting our mistakes and setting us back on a path towards achievement. As we get older we can take onboard new information and make adjustments ourselves. We need to get past the hurdle of being frustrated because we haven't got it right. Having gained insight into the need to EAT LESS *and* MOVE MORE, we must find the motivation to actually do it.

Here are some ideas. Pick something that has worked for you and suits your personality. Try several things until something helps. Ask God for insight and wisdom about this crucial area of motivation.

TARGETS

Are you the type of person who is motivated by targets, or just stressed by them? If you are motivated by them get on and set yourself targets. Be realistic so that you can be successful.

Has this helped in the past?	
Could it help now?	

EVENT

Some people find it helpful to look forward to an event and plan to be a dress size smaller for it. If that's you then stick the invitation on the fridge door! Remember to be realistic so that you can be successful.

Has this helped in the past?	
Could it help now?	

COMPETITIVE

If you like competition, challenge someone else to follow this plan and compete for points. Set up a point scheme like one for a pound lost and one for a kilometre walked or rowed or cycled. Be determined to win.

Has this helped in the past?	
Could it help now?	

PARTNERSHIP

Agree with another person that you will both follow the plan and encourage each other. Think about doing it for yourself and the other person. Be honest and be accountable. Exercise together, eat together, unpack your burdens together, pray together. Be determined that you are both going to succeed. Pick each other up when you fall.

Has this helped in the past?	
Could it help now?	

SPONSORSHIP

Why not raise money for a good cause, or in memory of a loved one? If that would keep you motivated then go out there and get your sponsors. Contact local businesses and your local paper. Tell everyone you are doing it, so you can't duck out.

Has this helped in the past?	
Could it help now?	

JUSTICE

There is enough food in this world for everyone. Yet some people have too little and others of us have too much. If you want to do something about this situation you can. Start by changing your own eating and drinking and giving the money you save to feed the hungry. Don't get stuck in the guilt rut, do something about it!

Has this helped in the past?	
Could it help now?	

NEW START

Starting, or renewing, a relationship with God can be very motivational. A whole new beginning. Seeing ourselves as God sees us can be a revelation. Awaken your spirituality and move forward with God.

Has this helped in the past?	
Could it help now?	

HEALTH

Big people are heading downhill towards diabetes, cancer, heart disease, joint problems and immobility at a much faster rate than their smaller friends. You can move yourself further back up the hill if you choose to EAT LESS *and* MOVE MORE. Is your health important to you?

Has this helped in the past?	
Could it help now?	

FAMILY

Focus on the children amongst your family and friends. Do you want to see them grow up? If you have a strong desire to see your Grandchildren grow up you could use that to motivate you to change your health status. If you are hoping to start a family it will be helpful to get your eating under control.

Has this helped in the past?	
Could it help now?	

GROUP SUPPORT

Taking part in a support group has been shown to be one of the most helpful motivational activities available. Shared experience, information exchange, and encouragement help to keep everyone on track.

Has this helped in the past?	
Could it help now?	

SUMMARY

The Simplest Diet Ever

EAT LESS *and* MOVE MORE

Let's stop saving up for a rainy day, and instead spend more. We do this by eating less than our body needs, and by moving our bodies more.

This is not a quick fix. This is gradual change that will make a difference in the long term. Start with one day a week and increase that to two days when you feel ready. Stay with this until you are ready to move up to three days, and so on up to five days a week. Remember to do both things, eating less and moving more.

Few of us can successfully deal with our eating issues until we have dealt with our life issues. That's why we need to be looking at our hearts, minds and spirits as well as our bodies.

We are not looking to dwell in the past but to move forward. We have to move on from where we are and not from where we would like to be. We can't alter our past, but we can take control of how it affects us now.

When we focus on how we feel about ourselves we get stuck in a rut. The value in approaching our food issues in a holistic way is that it doesn't just look at our body, or how we feel. It leads us towards the healing of our hearts. It walks us towards God and when we start to focus, not on what we feel about ourselves, but on what he thinks about us, we can get out of that rut.

My reasons to stay the same
Reasons to **EAT LESS** *and* **MOVE MORE**
Which day are you going to start?

www.simplestever.me.uk

FEEDBACK
If you have found this book helpful and would like to share with others how the Simplest Diet Ever has affected your life please send an account, with your contact details, to the author via the website   www.simplestever.me.uk
        or by email   Feedback@simplestever.me.uk

OTHER USEFUL WEBSITES

Information about faith
www.rejesus.co.uk
www.christianity.org.uk

Counselling available in the UK
www.acc-uk.org
www.bacp.co.uk

Diets and slimming clubs

www.glycemicindex.com

www.low-carbdiet.co.uk

www.Weightwatchers.co.uk

www.LighterLife.com

www.slimmingworld.com

www.caloriecontrol.org

www.gidiet.com

www.thedietplate.co.uk

www.tescodiets.com

www.slim-fast.com

www.weighdown.com

www.rosemaryconley.com

Health
www.verity-pcos.org.uk (Polycystic ovary disease)
www.pwsa.co.uk   (Prader-Willi Syndrome)
www.heartuk.org.uk   (The Cholesterol charity)
www.thyroiduk.org
www.diabetes.org.uk
www.cancerresearchuk.org

www.ingramcontent.com/pod-product-compliance
Lightning Source LLC
Chambersburg PA
CBHW030029290326
41934CB00005B/555